*Ancient Natural Beauty
Secrets!*

Natural Beauty

*Organic Superfoods, Essential
Oils, Natural Remedies,
Homemade Beauty Recipes,
Skin Care Secrets, And More
Tips For Anti-Aging And
Youthful Appearance!*

I0428310

Sarah Brooks

STOP!!! Before you read any further....Would you like to know the secrets of Anti-Aging?

If your answer is yes, then you are not alone. Thousands of people are looking for the secret to reducing wrinkles, looking younger, and maintaining a youthful appearance.

If you have been searching for these answers without much luck, you are in the right place!

Not only will you gain incredible insight in this book, but because I want to make sure to give you as much value as possible, right now for a limited time you can get full **100% FREE access to a VIP bonus eBook** entitled **Anti-Aging Made Easy!**

Just Go Here For Free Instant Access:

www.LuxyLifeNaturals.com

Legal Notice

Disclaimer Notice

Table Of Contents

Introduction

I want to thank you and congratulate you for purchasing the book, *"Natural Beauty: Ancient Natural Beauty Secrets! Organic Superfoods, Essential Oils, Natural Remedies, Homemade Beauty Recipes, Skin Care Secrets, And More Tips For Anti-Aging And Youthful Appearance!"*

This book contains proven steps and strategies on how to stay youthful through the years with the use of ancient but effective natural beauty remedies. This book also teaches you the essentials in staying beautiful and glowing through simple steps that you can do at home without spending a dime. This is a must-read for people who are aspiring to maintain their good looks in practical, risk-free and natural ways.

Thanks again for purchasing this book, I hope you enjoy it!

Chapter 1: Ancient Natural Beauty Secrets – What Are They?

Beauty concerns are universal. They've been and will remain an issue for the human race regardless of any age, gender or era. Can you imagine how people in the past managed to survive these beauty dilemmas?

People who lived in the ancient times have found their own ways to achieve ageless beauty. They were curious, driven and brave enough to experiment with their only resource – nature. Luckily for mankind, nature has all the answers. Take a sneak peek at these ancient beauty secrets!

Beauty tips and tricks come and go; they rise and fall according to the latest beauty trends. However, there are some beauty secrets which stood the test of time. These classic beauty secrets have proven themselves to be more resilient than a beauty hype that everybody forgets after a week and that is simply because they deliver on their promises consistently.

But what's so good about these ancient beauty secrets that would get you dying to try and stick to them for good? Here are some of them:

• Ancient beauty solutions are natural

Going back to the past might be helpful when it comes to beauty ideas. The pureness of the materials they use back then (when there was nothing but nature to turn to) is simply too good to forget. There were no harmful chemicals to speak of, only pure natural goodness.

Ancient beauty solutions are raw

Our elders did not care much about product processing. Without the technological breakthroughs during that time, you cannot really expect their beauty products to be as carefully processed as the products sold in the market today. This would only mean one thing – ancient beauty remedies are made from nothing less than raw and roughly processed materials in its purest and most natural state. As such, it retains most of the natural goodness that it contains which would otherwise be stripped off by product processing.

•   Ancient beauty solutions do not trigger harmful effects
These ancient secrets are made of pure natural goodness which causes little or no harm at all to the body. This would mean fewer health concerns and worry about the things you're putting in your body. By using natural beauty remedies, you can always have the peace of mind knowing that you can get beautiful without compromising your health.

•   Ancient beauty solutions are usually cheap and even FREE!
Ancient beauty treats are all good news for anyone who wants to get beautiful on a budget. The good thing about these ancient beauty items is that most of them can be found in your backyard or kitchen. They don't always have to be in an expensive salon or spa that you can't afford to go to every single time a pimple or two pops out. All of these lead us to believe in one thing: *you can never put a price on beauty!*

Chapter 2: Organic Superfoods – Healthy Food Choices For A Younger You

People who lived during the ancient days are considerably known to have a longer lifespan than the people living today. In fact, these ancient people can live up to a hundred years and still remain physically fit and beautiful. Ever wonder why that is? The secret is simple and still true nowadays – they eat nothing but organic super foods.

What are these organic super foods that can help you attain ageless beauty and health? Here are some of them:

1. Salmon

Common among dieters, Salmon is a super food that can help you attain healthy hair, skin and nails. Aside from being a delicious meal that can keep you full for hours, Salmon is rich in Omega-3 fatty acids, iron, Vitamin B-12 and good fats. 2-3 servings of Salmon can help you get most of your essential fatty acids requirement in a day.

2. Acai Berries and Pomegranates

These red-colored fruits have anti-oxidant properties which can help protect you from all sorts of diseases, including skin infections. They can also help your skin look younger by fighting off free radicals which causes premature and rapid aging. They likewise promote good blood flow to the skin, making skin regeneration easier and faster.

3. Kiwis, Mangoes and Oranges

High Vitamin C content is the common denominator of all these citrus fruits. Aside from its good taste, these fruits actually help keep your gums and teeth strong. Furthermore, these fruits can help you satisfy your sweet tooth because of its sweet, tangy flavor. No need for you to crave for sugary and unhealthy snacks anymore!

Vitamin C also promotes the production of collagen, a tissue known to improve skin elasticity and texture.

4. Flaxseeds

These little seeds are recommended if you want your skin to be smooth and acne-free! Acne breakouts are oftentimes the result of hormonal imbalance due to lack of proper nutrient supply in the body. Flaxseeds contain high amounts of Omega fatty acids which help balance estrogen levels, thus preventing hormonal imbalance which causes abnormal weight gain, mood swings and acne breakouts.

5. Berries

Feeling bloated and puffy? If so, berries are all you need to get all that extra fluid out of your body! Berries are packed with natural antioxidants, Vitamin C, Potassium and minerals which can help you balance everything in your system, including hormones and excess fluid. With its high antioxidant content, this super food is sure to help you deal with the signs of aging too!

Berries, being a delicious super food can easily be incorporated in your meal. You can eat it as a dessert or you can make a smoothie for breakfast. Either way, eating berries would help you remain full longer and curb your sweet tooth.

Who says eating healthy and staying young is difficult? With these super foods, all you have to do is sit back and enjoy delicious yet nutrient-packed snacks!

Chapter 3: Essential Oils For Beauty That Shines

Then and now, essential oils have been a beauty staple that never goes out of trend. They are very much used as an ingredient in moisturizers because of its rich, soothing and moisturizing properties. Take a look at some of the essential oils used by people then and now to attain a natural and ageless beauty that shines!

1) Sunflower Oil

   Sunflower oil is derived from sunflower seed extracts which are a rich source of Vitamin E. The benefits of this essential oil have already been recognized around the world and here are some of them:

   a) Lightens scars and unwanted marks on the body

   b) Moisturizes the face, hair and nails

   c) Act as eye moisturizer to lighten eye circles and minimize eye puffing

   d) Soothes skin irritation and insect bites

   e) Act as overall body moisturizer gentle enough even for people with sensitive skin

   f) Serves as make up remover

   With all these benefits at hand, you wouldn't go wrong with a bottle or two of this miracle oil. The good news is that sunflower is abundant, so its by-products including its oil are sold in the market at affordable prices.

2) Baobab Oil

Baobab Oil is an essential oil derived from the seeds of the Baobab tree. This tree, though may be found in other parts of the world, is native to Africa. In Africa, this oil was first used in the ancient times for the treatment of muscle aches and rheumatism. However, other uses for this oil have been discovered. In Zambia, Africa people used this oil during bath for babies, noting its moisturizing and cleansing property mild enough to take care of sensitive baby skin. Later on, it became a beauty staple used to help maintain skin elasticity and regeneration very much needed to maintain an ageless face.

3) Camellia Oil

To have that ageless beauty, a healthy hair is a must. Remember that it is not only the skin and the face that you should be wary of because hair as the crowning glory can make or break your appearance. The next question is, how do you maintain healthy hair? Camellia Oil can help you in that department!

Camellia Oil is an essential oil used by Japanese women in order to keep their hair sleek and healthy. Camellia Oil has high oleic acids, protein and glycerides content which is perfect for nourishing the hair. The oil is potent enough to allow you to get rid of your usual hot oil treatment. Just put a teaspoon of Camellia Oil to cover your hair, put on a hot towel for 20 to 30 minutes and you're as good as salon-pampered!

4) Tea Tree Oil

Pimples and blemishes are among the most common facial problems that people have nowadays thanks to the polluted environment and chemical-laden products. With all the dirt in the surroundings, it is not surprising that most people find it hard to maintain a clear and smooth face.

Old people have had the same problems and most would tell you they managed it using nothing but Tea Tree Oil. Tea Tree Oil has rich anti-oxidant properties to help the face get rid of dirt and impurities which cause acne breakout. It is also rich in other vitamins to help keep your face smooth, elastic and clean all the time.

5) Chamomile Oil

One of the major causes of premature aging is stress. Inevitable as it is, there are other ways on how to diffuse stress and keep your beauty. One of the ancient ways to do it is through aroma therapy, and undoubtedly Chamomile Oil is the perfect partner for such.

Chamomile Oil has a very relaxing scent which can help your mind and body release tension. It also has moisturizing properties that can help your skin stay fresh and hydrated. Just put some drops onto your bathtub and watch it work wonders as it relaxes your mind and moisturize your skin.

Grab these must-have natural oils for a beautiful and younger you! These oils are nothing but natural, making them far safer than mineral oil - a harmful chemical that most commercial moisturizers have. Remember that your skin deserves only the best and the purest!

Chapter 4: Natural Remedies For Wrinkles

Wrinkles are probably one of the first signs of aging that people hate so much. It doesn't only make your skin crease but it also makes your appearance look less radiant. But don't fret yet! There are easy and effective ways on how to combat wrinkles. Below are some of the natural remedies for wrinkles that you can use:

- Egg white and Lemon Face mask

    How to do it:

    Prepare 1 egg and 1 medium-sized lemon. Separate the egg white from the yolk and set it aside. In the meantime, squeeze half a lemon to get its juice and mix it with the egg white. Mix properly. Put the mixture on your face for 10 – 15 minutes. Rinse it off completely with water.

    Benefits of this face mask:

    Egg whites are known to have wrinkle-fighting properties because of their concentrated protein content. It provides a much needed protein supply for the wrinkled skin to make it look and feel firmer. On the other hand, lemon is very rich in Vitamin C which helps your skin fight off bacteria and skin infections. Together, this face mask combination will help you have firm and smooth skin.

- Olive Oil and Oatmeal Face Mask

  How to do it:

  Prepare 2 teaspoon of olive oil and ½ cup of oatmeal. In a bowl, put in the oatmeal and add the olive oil. Mix and mash the ingredients together until it becomes creamy. If it's not creamy enough to stick, add some more oil.

  Benefits of this face mask:

  Oatmeal is known to be a good source of protein and fiber which can also be beneficial to the skin. It fights off germs to make sure that your skin is clear and it serves as a natural exfoliant to ward off dead skin cells. Meanwhile, olive oil serves as skin moisturizer to protect the skin from being too dry after the exfoliation process.

- Aloe Vera and Rosehip Oil Face Mask

  How to do it:

  Snip one Aloe Vera leaf (if you have it) or get some Aloe Vera essence elsewhere. Rosehip oil is often processed, so you have to get it at a nearby organic beauty store.

  If you're using Aloe Vera leaf, just cut it into 2 and apply the juice directly to your face. Leave it on for 10 minutes and rinse. Afterwards, apply rosehip oil all over your face, leave it on for 10 – 15 minutes and rinse off.

Benefits of this face mask:

Aloe Vera is nature's best cure for minor skin problems like allergy, irritation, acne and blemishes. It cleanses the skin thoroughly and leaves the skin smooth and blemish-free, making it a good primer before applying rosehip oil. Rosehip oil on the other hand, is said to reverse wrinkle formation as it soothes and moisturize the skin, making it one of the most coveted ingredients in the cosmetic industry when it comes to anti-aging products.

Say goodbye to wrinkles with the use of these natural remedies! These natural face masks are easily accessible and affordable so you won't have any reason to put up with those creases.

Chapter 5: Ancient Beauty Must-Haves

To stay beautiful and ageless, people who lived in the old days considered some beauty staples as a must-have. Ever wonder what those things are? Take a peek at some of them!

- Flour Corn (also known as blue corn)

  For hundreds of years, Native American tribes like Hopi, Zuni and Navajo have relied on flour corn not only for food and religious rituals but also for its beauty enhancement properties.

  Blue corn (the other name for flour corn) is coarser than yellow corn and is primarily used for making flour or cornmeal. Aside from that, ground flour corn was also used by natives as a skin cleanser and purifier. It was rubbed to the skin before the start of rituals and ceremonies, on the belief that it could rinse off impurities. It acts as skin exfoliant, ridding the skin of dead skin cells and promoting faster cell regeneration. Because it was easily accessible especially for farmers, people of the tribes always carry a bag or two of this beauty must have.

- Fireweed

  Before contemporary winter coats have been tailored, people back then used animal skin and fireweed to protect their skin from the cold. The root of the fireweed plant is dried, powdered and stored up as a winter must have. The powdered fireweed is rubbed into the skin for protection against the harsh effects of the cold.

- Saw Palmetto

  Back when hormonal imbalance wasn't a common knowledge, native people used Saw Palmetto to get rid of facial hair in women who are experiencing high testosterone levels. As studies now suggest, Saw Palmetto helps regulate excessive hair growth by effectively suppressing DHT production (testosterone derived) in the body.

- Sweet grass

  Considered as sacred, this flat-leafed bladed grass was used to purify both individuals and surroundings. As a beauty regimen though, it was used to treat windburn and dry skin. Some people also boil it to make a tea to be used as hair tonic and body fragrance.

- Wild Mint

  Cheyenne Indians have been using wild mint as hair oil for quite a long time now. Wild mint has anti-inflammatory properties that help the scalp and hair remain itch-free. In addition to that, Thompson Indians also used Wild Mint tonic for hair dressing purposes.

- Yucca

  Baldness and thinning hair are also prominent signs of aging. One of the ways people in the old days handled the same is with the use of Yucca plant. The roots of the Yucca plant were crushed and used as hair wash for balding people and newborns alike to help promote hair growth.

Native people have nothing but nature to rely on when it comes to their beauty needs. However, this didn't stop them from being beautiful with these natural secrets! As modern as today is, it wouldn't hurt to try these ancient secrets, would it?

Chapter 6: Skin Care Secrets To A Youthful Glow

Not contented with your skin? Do you feel like you can have a better skin than what you have? That's perfectly fine because you're ahead of the game. In fact, most people take their skin for granted and just wait for their skin to look old enough before they even bother to care.

A glowing skin can be attained in two ways: by *doing* some things and by *avoiding* others. Listed are the dos and don'ts for a skin that glows!

What to do:

- Relieve stress through aromatherapy

- Go natural and avoid chemical-laden products as much as possible

- Eat healthy

- Exercise for at least 20 minutes a day

- Get ample sleep (at least 6-8 hours of sound and deep sleep)

What *not* to do:

- Smoke cigarettes

- Drink too much liquor

- Sleep with make up on

- Expose yourself to the sun for long periods of time

As much as people should know what they should do, it is sometimes knowing what they should avoid that makes the total difference. Now that you know both, you are now one step closer to your goal!

Chapter 7: Surprising Anti-Aging Solutions You Never Knew Existed

There are beauty secrets that you often hear about while there are some that you never even knew existed. These are uncommon, never-heard-of natural beauty remedies that will surprise you up a bit until you discover the wonders that they can do for your body. Read on to know more about these exotic beauty secrets!

1. Rooibos

   Rooibos is a plant exclusively found in Cape Town, South Africa. The leaves of this plant were made into a red bush tea used both as an anti-allergen and an antioxidant. The essence of the tea has been used to treat skin conditions such as eczema, dermatitis, rashes and inflammation.

2. Pearl Powder

   Pearl powder is an ancient Chinese secret to beautiful skin. It is made of crushed and powdered oyster shells and is known to contain essential amino acids to rejuvenate the skin. More often than not, pearl powder is used together with a mixture of honey and egg yolk so treat inflammation and soothe skin irritations.

3. Cactus

   Who knew cactus have anti-aging properties? This prickly pear contains a lot of nutrients such as

Riboflavin, B12, Vitamin A and Vitamin D, all known to nourish the skin and halt aging. Overall, it helps increase skin elasticity and speeds up cell regeneration.

4. Persimmon

Want to be as flawless as a geisha? Persimmon might just be the magic you're looking for! This is exactly the Japanese beauty secret dating back in the geisha days. Persimmon is a Japanese fruit containing a lot of vitamins and minerals like phosphorous, magnesium and iodine. Persimmon is often combined with whipped cream before it is applied to the face to help create a flawless complexion.

These exotic beauty ingredients may not be always accessible, but still it's good to know and experiment a little with your beauty regimen from time to time. Go ahead and try some of these exciting beauty recipes when you feel like it!

Chapter 8: Proven Ways To Maintain A Youthful Look

Having a youthful glow can be achieved almost instantly with all the cosmetic procedures available nowadays. In fact, you can immediately have a glowing skin right after you did a facial treatment for as short as 15 minutes. However, the real challenge lies in keeping your appearance healthy in the long haul and without much reliance on cosmetic procedures. To be able to do that, you need to build a good beauty regimen to practice over the years. Here are some quick tips on how you could maintain a youthful appearance:

- Brighten up your wardrobe

  Your wardrobe can tell so much about you. It can tell much about your style, preferences, even your age. If your wardrobe consist mostly sweats, pants and boring clothes, it's no wonder that you look way beyond your age. It's now time for you to spice up your wardrobe!

  To look young, your must dress like you are indeed young. The fact that you're getting older doesn't mean that you can't be trendy and stylish. There are so many ways to look younger when you dress up; you just have to be explore a little. For starters, get rid of those plain dark tops and dresses. You can do much better than wear funeral attire. Opt for light colored dresses and do not be all covered up. Show a bit of skin and know what your physical assets are.

- Exfoliate and moisturize

  Sometimes, the skin looks aged because of the dead skin cells lurking around your body. These are old layers of the skin which turns dark and needs to be exfoliated from time to time. You have to know that the body goes through natural exfoliation but the process can take long. As such, it wouldn't hurt for you to help in the natural exfoliating process by using exfoliants such as body scrubs and salts. However, don't forget to moisturize right after exfoliating because your body loses its natural moisture in the process.

  Putting on moisturizer is also a must for young-looking skin. Dry skin tends to patch up easily, making it prone to itch and skin irritations. While the body has natural moisture, factors like sun exposure, stress, and long bath time can take it away, leaving your skin dry. Always bring a moisturizer with you so your skin is sure to stay hydrated all the time!

- Relax once in a while

  Stress is probably one of the main causes of premature aging. While stress is an inevitable part of life, you shouldn't let it get in the way of looking and feeling younger. Give yourself a break and relax those fine lines for a while! This will help your body cope with all the strains and pressure of life. You deserve it!

- Laugh every chance you get

  Laugh lines are surely better than wrinkles. By laughing, you release some of the tension in your body, making you feel lighter and happier. Science would also tell you that smiling uses far less face muscles than frowning, so it helps your facial muscles relax a bit. Most importantly, laughing takes away 10 years off your age by making you look radiant and problem-free!

Being youthful isn't all about being young in age; it's more about being young at heart. Nourish yourself as an individual in all aspects in your life and that youthful appearance will surely follow!

Chapter 9: The Anti-Aging Benefits Of Honey And Coconut Oil

Almost every beauty secret makes mention of these two very potent gifts of nature – honey and coconut. Both of them have anti-aging properties which can cure almost every aging problem there is. Continue reading to discover more about these miracle ingredients!

Honey:

Raw honey is known for its antibacterial properties. It keeps the face clean enough to ward off infections, acne breakouts and blemishes. It also has antioxidants which helps fight off free radicals that destroy healthy cells in the body.

Honey is also a good cure for people who are suffering from large pores because of its clarifying properties. Honey goes down to unclog the pores of dirt and grime and leaves the skin clear. Honey can be used directly on the face as mask or you may also combine it with lemon.

Coconut Oil:

Coconut oil on the other hand, is one of nature's most powerful moisturizers. It is also said to protect the skin from the harmful rays of the sun. Coconut oil is mainly composed of saturated fat, Vitamin E and protein which are the essentials for keeping your hair, scalp, skin, nails and body moisturized. This is also one of the safest natural products since very few are reported to have experienced adverse effects to it.

The good news about these natural cures is that they are available almost everywhere. You can drop by any grocery store and find one (at an affordable price too).

Chapter 10: Looking Ten Years Younger And Feeling Good About It!

After reading 9 chapters of this book, you are surely excited to try all of the stuff you read. Fortunately for you, that is the way forward to a younger and healthier you!

However, all the things that you've learned so far still have to be taken under several considerations. You cannot just jump in without knowing certain things. Here are the final considerations that you need to think about before making any changes to your beauty regimen:

- Health concerns/issues

  Your present health condition should be your primary consideration when making any changes on your diet and regimen. Of course, the changes that you will make should suit, or at least be harmless to your health. After all, what good is it if it's going to just make you ill?

  Always seek the advice of your doctor prior to any changes especially if you have a sensitive condition, i.e. pregnant, lactating, etc. This will give you the peace of mind you need.

- Allergic triggers

  The common misconception is that if it's natural, no skin irritation whatsoever can occur. This is completely wrong! Allergic reactions can occur to anyone, no matter how pure and natural the products they use are. For example, some people are naturally allergic to milk (lactose intolerant), mint and shrimp. Because of that, you have to know the contents of what you are putting in your body as well as your allergic triggers. If you have a history of allergic reaction to honey or coconut oil, might as well stop using them even though it has great anti-aging properties. The good news is that there are other alternatives that you may use on your skin. You just have to find what suits you best.

- Time and budget

  Time and budget are also considerations that you should take into account. Most of the time, the natural products aren't as easily accessible as the commercial ones so you really have to make an effort in finding them. Just keep in mind that it will be worth it in the end!

- Proper mindset

  The last and more important thing is to have the proper mindset. Feeling young and beautiful is not always about having a youthful appearance (although that is important too). Sometimes, you just need to be in the proper state of mind to feel really content and happy about yourself and no amount of makeover can be better than that. Just make sure that whatever you do, you do it because you want to and not because you want to please other people. After all, it is your life and it is you who will make the effort and reap the consequences.

You are now primed and ready to step ten years younger than your age! Go explore and discover all the things life has to offer as you feel more energized, healthier and younger!

Conclusion

Thank you again for purchasing the book *"Natural Beauty: Ancient Natural Beauty Secrets! Organic Superfoods, Essential Oils, Natural Remedies, Homemade Beauty Recipes, Skin Care Secrets, And More Tips For Anti-Aging And Youthful Appearance!"*

I am extremely excited to pass this information along to you, and I am so happy that you now have read and can hopefully implement these strategies going forward.

I hope this book was able to help you understand the different ways to pamper your body using natural recipes and how to maintain an ageless beauty throughout the years.

The next step is to get started using this information and to hopefully live a healthy, satisfying and happy life!

Please don't be someone who just reads this information and doesn't apply it, the strategies in this book will only benefit you if you use them!

If you know of anyone else that could benefit from the information presented here please inform them of this book.

Finally, if you enjoyed this book and feel it has added value to your life in any way, please take the time to share your thoughts and post a review on Amazon. It'd be greatly appreciated!

Thank you and good luck!

Preview Of:

Ultimate Coconut Oil Guide!

<u>Coconut Oil</u>

Coconut Oil Recipes For Organic Skin Care And Natural Beauty, Clean Eating For Weight Loss, Shinning Hair, Better Brain Function And Overall Health!

Introduction

I want to thank you and congratulate you for purchasing the book, *Coconut Oil: Ultimate Coconut Oil Guide! - Coconut Oil Recipes For Organic Skin Care And Natural Beauty, Clean Eating For Weight Loss, Shining Hair, Better Brain Function And Overall Health!*

This book contains proven steps and strategies on how you can take full advantage of the beauty, weight loss and health benefits that coconut oil has to offer. Through this book, you will learn more about:

1. What makes coconut oil healthy?
2. How it can help you get better, more glowing skin.
3. Its effects on your hair and making healthier.
4. Can coconut oil improve your brain function?
5. Weight loss benefits and how it can boost your metabolism.
6. Coconut oil and how it can help treat different illnesses.
7. Recipes for both your diet as well as organic skin care.
8. How to choose the right coconut oil for your needs.

We hope that through this book, you'll be able to recognize the amount of potential that a single bottle of coconut oil contains.

Thanks again for purchasing this book, I hope you enjoy it!

Chapter 1: Coconut Oil For Natural Beauty And Health

These days, more and more people are becoming aware of the effects that chemically manufactured products has on their bodies. As such, many of them have turned to a greener, more organic lifestyle that advocates going all natural when it comes to their food as well as the different products that they use on their bodies.

This isn't surprising, of course, considering the fact that there are a number of illnesses which are associated with constant use of synthetic and often chemical-laden skin and health products. There are certain risks that one must bear when using it; risks which can be avoided altogether if one were to switch over to something that's a bit closer to nature.

The coconut oil is a favorite among health buffs as it is one of those by-products that can be used in a multitude of ways. On one hand, it can be eaten and taken as a supplement which would boost your overall health. On the other, it can be applied topically and used as a beauty product as well as a means of treating certain skin issues.

You get all of these benefits but without worrying about its harmful effects to the body.

Why is it considered one of the best natural remedies out there?

It's all in the composition. About 99% of it is composed of saturated fats (which, in this case isn't as bad as it sounds) as well as traces of polyunsaturated fatty acids and monosaturated fatty acids. Virgin coconut oil retains a higher amount of the good stuff thus it is also valued higher.

It also contains lauric acid and quite a generous amount of it at that. When digested by the body, this would turn into monolaurin and is very beneficial when it comes to dealing with different bacteria and viruses. Diseases such as influenza and herpes are just two of the things that coconut oil can cure in a jiff. A tablespoon of it a day keeps the doctor away, so to speak.

Besides these, it is also one of the most powerful inhibitors of quite a number of different pathogenic organisms ranging from your usual viruses to even protozoa. All of this, of course, is attributed to its high lauric acid content.

For beauty and skincare

Coconut can also be used for cosmetic or skin care purposes. We'll get to the specifics of this in later chapters but to quickly summarize, it is often used for: Hair care, skin care, nails, lips as well as treating different skin issues such as psoriasis. It helps keep the skin youthful and glowing as well as protect it from harmful UV rays.

Thanks for Previewing My Exciting Book Entitled:

"Coconut Oil: Ultimate Coconut Oil Guide! Coconut Oil Recipes For Organic Skin Care And Natural Beauty, Clean Eating For Weight Loss, Shinning Hair, Better Brain Function And Overall Health!"

To purchase this book, simply go to the Amazon Kindle store and simply search:

"COCONUT OIL"

Then just scroll down until you see my book. You will know it is mine because you will see my name "Sarah Brooks" underneath the title.

Alternatively, you can visit my author page on Amazon to see this book and other work I have done. Thanks so much, and please don't forget your free bonuses

DON'T LEAVE YET! - CHECK OUT YOUR FREE BONUSES BELOW!

Free Bonus Offer: Get Free Access To The www.LuxyLifeNaturals.com VIP Newsletter!

Once you enter your email address you will immediately get free access to this awesome newsletter!

But wait, right now if you join now for free you will also get free access to the "Anti-Aging Made Easy" free EBook!

To claim both your FREE VIP NEWSLETTER MEMBERSHIP and your FREE BONUS Ebook on ANTI-AGING MADE EASY!

Just Go To:

www.LuxyLifeNaturals.com